Neurological Series

I0397040

Fibromyalgia
and
Chronic Fatigue

PAIN
ACHE
HURT
DISCOMFORT
STRESS
ANXIETY
FEAR
DOUBT
WORRY
DEPRESSION
GLUME
HOPELESS
BRAIN FOG
DESPAIR
BLUE

JC Spencer

?

Is Fibromyalgia and Chronic Fatigue
caused by something?

or

Is Fibromyalgia and Chronic Fatigue
caused by lack of something?

ISBN 978-1545563502

Glycoscience Mini-Book Series is
an educational project of
GlycoScience Institute, Inc.
PO Box 73089 – Houston, Texas 77273

Inquires for lecture bookings at universities,
fund-raising, and other events,
The author may be reached at
jcs@endowmentmed.org

Content

Chapter One

Chapter Two

Chapter Three

Chapter Four

"Where there is no vision, the people perish..."
Proverbs 29:18a KJV

Foreword

Into his third decade JC Spencer has participated with many M.D.s, PhDs, researchers and educators in several countries and has written reports on hundreds of laboratory, anecdotal, and clinical results.

After founding The Endowment for Medical Research in Houston, Texas, in 2002, it sponsored Glycoscience Medical Conferences. The major aim of these very successful and well attended Conferences was to educate healthcare workers and others of the new scientific area of Glycoscience and its possible application to helping individuals who suffer from poor health especially chronic neurodegenerative conditions.

Fibromyalgia and Chronic Fatigue has brought suffering pain and neurological dysfunction to millions. Researchers have learned that the neurological implications is caused by or accentuated by a misfolding of the proteins on the surface of human cells. We have learned through Glycoscience how to better fold the proteins.

Knowledge of the nutritional damage that sugars and sweeteners have on the human body has blinded many scientists and researchers from seeing the beneficial sugars the body requires. The study of these various sugars is Glycoscience and the author coined the expression, "Smart Sugars."

The author has extensive studies and experiences covering more than two decades. He has uncovered a myriad of fascinating research concerning neurons. Our medical systems and all healthcare will benefit greatly as we better understand neurons and neurotransmitters. His studies include optimal nutrition for the brain and a host of relevant matters on basic psychology, savants, mental exercises and recovery from brain damage.

With his fellow pioneers in Glycoscience, he learned the benefits of a variety of collaborating disciplines that include pH, electrolytes, rogue electrons, mitochondria, and nutrition to name a few.

The TEXAS ENDOWMENT FOR MEDICAL RESEARCH in 2017 obtained a licensing agreement for intellectual properties and technologies and intellectual properties of earlier works consolidated with that from other organizations.

Introduction

If you have fibromyalgia, you probably have experienced times when you developed a craving for more sugar. It is as if sugar feeds fibromyalgia and chronic fatigue. The body cries out for more energy and a sugar spike may be a "Fix" for the moment.

The "Sugar Pill"

The "Sugar Pill" used as a placebo indicates just how worthless is regular sugar. But, it may be worse than that. Regular table sugar participates in causing or compounding fibromyalgia and chronic fatigue

In Chapter Three, I discuss a beneficial category of biological sugars. These sugars found in nature can actually save and extend your life. I have named them "Smart Sugars." Who would have thought that the sugar has the potential to solve some of our greatest health problems?

Smart Sugars are destined to take US to a better future. These sugars can provide healthier children and stressless parents. Studies verify that these special sugars can support neurological function for those with PTSÐ, MS, ALS, Parkinson's, Alzheimer's, Huntington's, Stroke, and other nerve function.

The special sugars are the building blocks for glycoforms. Glycoforms are glycan and glycoprotein signal receptor sites on the surface of your cells. Glycolipids operate inside your cells.

What Are Smart Sugars?
These Smart Sugars are operating this moment in your body as your cellular Operating System (OS). Their responsibility is to process all DNA data communication to function, maintain, repair, and replicate. These sugars actually give LIFE to your blood.

Glycoscience (glyco is Greek for sugar) has been hidden in plain sight and is now revealed to radically change how we live. Glycoscience IS the New Frontier of Medicine. This emerging technology will make a major difference in human health. It will do so because the sugars instigate an aggressive attack on viral infections and resistant bacteria.

Big Pharma and our government have already invested billions of dollars in Glycoscience and the general public is still in the dark.

Knowledge of Glycoscience is young. The term "glycobiology" was coined at Oxford University in 1988.

Early in the 21st century, the science of sugars was reconsidered by the *National Academy of Sciences*, the top scientific governmental body in Washington, DC. This prestigious group is made up of Nobel Prize winners and those nominated by Nobel Prize winners.

A distinguished panel of glycoscientists was commissioned for a collaborative effort to explore the future of Glycoscience. The National Research Council drew from the National Academies: the National Academy of Sciences, National Academy of Engineering, Institute of Medicine. The project was supported by National Institutes of Health, the National Science Foundation, U.S. Department of Energy, the Food and Drug Administration, and the Howard Hughes Medical Institute. Together, they were commissioned to develop the roadmap for the future of Glycoscience. By the close of 2012, the panel published its 200 page report *Transforming Glycoscience - A Road Map for the Future.* Here, they went on record, stating that:

> **"Glycans impact the structure/function of every living cell in humans, animals, and plants."**

The Academy expanded on the importance of the sugars, saying:

> **"Glycans play roles in almost every biological process and are involved in every major disease"**
> and
> **"Elimination of any single class of glycans from an organism results in death."**

Another indication of the importance of Glycoscience is found in the bowels of the National Library of Medicine where almost 700,000 references point to research already conducted on some of the most significant life changing biological sugars. The majority of these papers were published within the last few years.

The Truths in this book are self-evident!

Chapter One

What is Fibromyalgia and Chronic Fatigue?

Scientists are baffled

The medical stance on fibromyalgia is that there is no cure.
People diagnosed with fibromyalgia usually have it for life.
Normal procedure is a series of attempts to lessen the symptoms.
Some are able to minimize their symptoms with a combination of
exercise, physical therapy, relaxation, and learning which foods
contribute to the pain and suffering.

S cientists are baffled by the symptoms of fibromyalgia which are overlapping with other disorders. Similarities with chronic fatigue are quite evident.

New findings may help us improve diagnosis and address fibromyalgia and chronic fatigue. Doctors are confused with what to call which. Scientists have not determined the cause for fibromyalgia. Number of diagnoses show that more than ninety percent (90%) with the fibromyalgia are women. Many medical doctors are skeptic if fibromyalgia is real or not.

Those who suffer from fibromyalgia and/or chronic fatigue syndrome often feel extreme fatigue after exertion which does not improve much, if any, with sleep or rest.

Headaches and muscle pain are common. The ability to concentrate and think clearly may persist with the pain for years.

A commonality with ventrally every ailment of humankind is a compromised immune system. The lowering of the immune system often leads to further compromising factors especially with the endocrine system.

Compromising immune function results in lowering ability to fight viral infections and other neurological disorders.

Research provides evidence that fibromyalgia or chronic fatigue syndrome triggers or provides pathways to other diseases.

Source and References:
Expand Your Mind - Improve Your Brain   http://endowmentmed.org/content/view/826/106/

Change Your Sugar, Change Your Life   http://DiabeticHope.com

http://EzineArticles.com/?expert=JC_Spencer

© The Endowment for Medical Research   http://endowmentmed.org

Communication makes everything happen.

Chapter Two

Neural Communication's Role with Fibromyalgia and Chronic Fatigue

**Neural communication
is signaling between the neurons
throughout the nervous system.**

Common Cause Found For
All Neurodegenerative Disorders

We had over a hundred Fibromyalgia and Chronic Fatigue, Alzheimer's and Parkinson sufferers in our Pilot Surveys at The Endowment for Medical Research before we knew there was a common cause.

The growing family of neurodegenerative disorders is epidemic. The commonality is misfolded polypeptide chains which are toxic to the cell.

Toxicity in the cell is a major contributing factor to corruption of the signals the cells receive and transmit via their glycoprotein receptor sites. The question appears to be, "*Did the toxins cause the misfolding of the protein or did the misfolding generate the toxins.*" While the answer may be, "*Both*", one thing is for certain; was the corruption of the signals that caused and compounded the abnormality.

Scientists conclude that glycomics deal with sugars. (Genomics deal with genes and proteomics deal with proteins.)

Glycoscience is the science that will change the way we address healthcare. Specific saccharides are required for the cells to be healthy and communicate with distinctive signals. Signal corruption may cause neurological abnormalities that lead to manifestation of many health challenges.

Symptoms and similarities often confuse the issue and result in wrong diagnoses. Sometimes there are overlaps in names because different doctors or researchers find the same or a similar disease and names it after themselves as first to describe the disease, or they name it after their patient as perhaps the first to be diagnosed.

Proper folding of proteins in individuals with one or more of these dysfunctions may find health benefits by improving the folding of the proteins. We have already achieved significant benefits in individuals with many of some 500 neurological dysfunctions.

**The genome is believed to contain only
30% of the health biomarkers while the
glycome may contain the other 70%.**

**Much research is needed and this fact will
forever change medical practice for the better.**

Chapter Three

Glycoscience - Future of Medicine and Healthcare

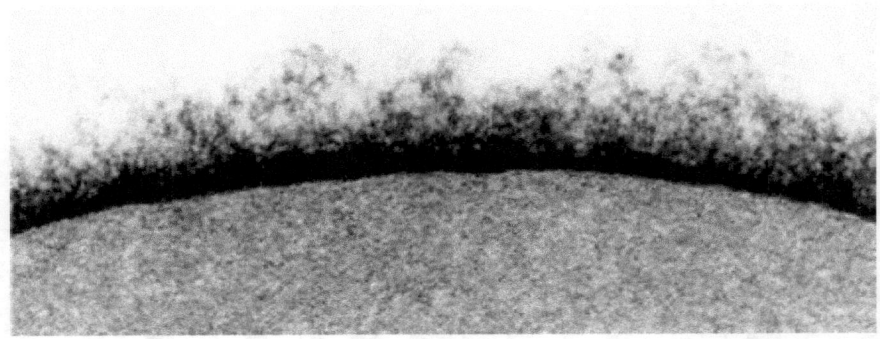

Glycan / Glycoproteins on the surface of a red blood cell. These Glycoforms transmit and receive all cellular signals for the human body.

Graphic used with permission: Source Voet and Voet

Glycobiology helps us better understand Fibromyalgia and Chronic Fatigue

The term "glycobiology" was coined in 1988 at Oxford University. Today, glycobiology explains that Cellular Communication is the key to all life.

Glycobiology is the foundational branch of Glycoscience that studies the essential sugars that are the building blocks of glycoforms.

Sugars are carbohydrates. Many carbohydrates are not good for your health. But, several specific sugars are so beneficial that they are essential to LIFE. They are at work in your body every moment. I call them Smart Sugars.

Glycans are links of specific sugar molecules.

DNA and proteins are formed by templates, while glycans are formed more from environmental influences. The cell's environmental factors contribute to each unique glycan design, as varied as fingerprints. These known and unknown factors provide each glycan with properties that are more complex and difficult to study and duplicate than genes.

Glycoproteins are links of specific protein with sugar molecules.

Specific glycans are attached to specific proteins. Structure and function are influenced by the DNA and cell environmental needs. Alignment of the glycans with the proteins determines cell function including blood type.

Glycolipids are links of specific sugar and lipid molecules:

Glycolipids provide cellular recognition and energy to help maintain membrane stability. This enables cells to attach to other cells to form tissue. Lipids contain hydrocarbons, the cellular building blocks for structure and function. Glycolipids are composed mostly of nonprotein cell membrane.

Glycans are the key to processing all communication and we are hardwired for...truth and perfection. Our cells are ever attempting to achieve purity by continuing to dump toxins out of the body.

Much of my writings and classes explore various aspects of Glycoscience and how cells communicate.

New Scientist, 10/02 reported, *"'This is going to be the future,'* declares biochemist Gerald Hart of Johns Hopkins University in Baltimore. *'We won't understand immunology, neurology, developmental biology or disease until we get a handle on glycobiology.'* ... *'If you ask, what is the glycome for a single cell type, it's probably many thousands of times more complex than the genome,'* says Ajit Varki, Director of the Glycobiology Research and Training Center at the University of California in San Diego ... Raymond Dwek, Head of the University of Oxford's Glycobiology Institute, who coined the term *"glycobiology"* in 1988, says that sugars were often dismissed as unimportant, *'as just decorations on proteins - people didn't know how to deal with them."* They could not have been more wrong.

As recent advances in genetics have unfolded, the importance of sugars has become ever more apparent ... Varki sees it as a journey of exploration. *'It's like we've just discovered the continent of North America. Now we have to send out scouting parties to find out how big it is ...'*

Many participants eating phytosugars (plant sugars), in our nutritional pilot surveys, not only experienced improved cognitive abilities, but also experienced overall general health and well being. If you are starting to replace your regular table sugar, we would appreciate your completing a general health evaluation form which you can request or download from our website at http://endowmentmed.org

While the science of glycobiology is relatively new it was not called as such until 1988. Some research in the US on glycoproteins and other sugar-containing molecules was conducted prior to 1980. In 1985 a research group at Oxford published a paper in *Nature* about glycosylation. Oxford University Press in 1988 started the journal *Glycobiology*. It was Raymond Dwek, Head of the University of Oxford's Glycobiology Institute, who actually coined the term "*glycobiology*" in 1988, and it was soon used in science around the world.

The following is a quote from the Institute for Glycomics at Griffith University: "*Glycomics is the study of applied biology and chemistry that deals with the structure and function of carbohydrates (sugars). The term glycomics is derived from the chemical prefix for sweetness or a sugar, 'glyco', and was formed to follow the naming convention established by genomics* (which deals with genes) *and proteomics* (which deals with proteins)."

Glycomics and genomics are shining lights in the field of medical science. These lights are a blinding force in the dark age of that region of medical science that limits itself to drug use and abuse.

Smart Sugars are the ingredients for tomorrow's healthcare system. The number of physicians integrating sugars into their practices is growing because they are witnessing remarkable results almost regardless of what is wrong with their patients. Maybe treating the symptom has not been the solution. Understanding the cause and using an ounce of prevention is worth a pound of cure.

Faulty and False Communication

When our cells have an abundance of healthy glycans coating the cellular transceivers, things work more effectively in the body. Simply stated, when we don't, things go awry. *We now know from the study of Glycoscience that every ailment, every disease, all sickness is the result of faulty communication.* Even a split second of non-communication or faulty communication during a baby's nine month gestation period can cause spina bifida deformities.

Faulty signals can render your immune system dysfunctional. It may become weak and ineffective, or confused and attack your own body's cells as an autoimmune disorder. Autoimmune and degenerative diseases involve missing sugars on the cell's surface.

Glycoscience teaches us that neuron transmission is damaged by manmade confusion that tangles communication. Information is often blocked completely or the wires are crossed to give a totally different message than intended. The earlier you start in life to build an excellent neurological transmission system the better.

False Signals Cause Chaos
that may manifest as Fibromyalgia

False signals, sooner or later, develop chaos. Lack of any communication is more trust worthy than miscommunication. False signals make it so you do not know where you are going and that is where you are likely to end up. Lack of communication simply stops all progress.

We have developed a pathway to improve brain function with Smart Sugars that are the building blocks for the Operating System (OS) of the brain and every cell of your body. Communication between cells is the responsibility of the Smart Sugars. However, the choice of morality, the choice of Truth is left up to the individual. Truth is hardwired into the brain.

When you go against Truth, your whole body knows and responds with a compounding stress level. Stress causes aging and the need to improve the immune system. Smart Sugars improve immunity and reduce stress.

Quality and quantity of Smart Sugars in the blood can be evaluated.

Major Find in 2011

In 2011, Dr. John Axford, past president of the Royal Society of Medicine, conducted an open label study to evaluate the safety and effects of ingesting certain Smart Sugars from plants, i.e., polysaccharides. The work of Dr. Axford and his team included in vitro and in vivo studies which suggest that certain saccharides have immunomodulatory effects and impact cellular glycosylation. Oral ingestion caused no adverse events and a significant overall shift toward increased sialyation*. Scientists have proved beyond a doubt, that these specific sugars are critical to life and health.

* **sialyation** *is not to be confused with sylation. Sialyation has to do with sialic acid, a generic term for a derivative of neuraminic acid, a monosaccharide. This Smart Sugar is commonly called N-acetylneuraminic acid and is found in glycoproteins. There is significant concentration of sialic acid in the human brain where it plays a role in neural transmission through the synapsis.*

sylation *has to do with the bonding of molecules. When the word "glyco" is placed in front of "sylation", it means to bond a sugar, i.e. glycosylation. When a specific sugar is bonded, the name of that sugar is placed in front of "sylation." To sylate mannose is mannosylation. To sylate fucose is called fucosylation.*

Glycoscience IS The Road Map for the Future

The top scientific governmental body in Washington, DC, the *National Academy of Sciences* (NAS), is made up of Nobel Prize winners or those nominated by Nobel Prize winners. This distinguished community appointed a panel to publish the 200 page report ***Transforming Glycoscience - A Road Map for the Future***. Here, they went on record in 2012 stating that: "*Glycans impact the structure/function of every living cell in humans, animals, and plants.*" The Academy expanded on the importance of the sugars saying: "*Glycans play roles in almost every biological process and are involved in every major disease*" and "*Elimination of any single class of glycans from an organism results in death.*"

To bring Glycoscience from the recently little known into the mainstream, *Transforming Glycoscience* recommends that all university and high school science departments teach Glycoscience.

The National Academies - NAS, National Academy of Engineering, Institute of Medicine, and National Research Council - consider this science so important that their 10-year goal includes, "*integrating Glycoscience into relevant disciplines in high school, undergraduate and graduate education, and developing curricula and standardized testing for science competency which would increase public as well as professional awareness.*"

The Future

Glycoscience's disruptive technology will forever change our medical system. The future of medicine will include cell regeneration, neurodegenerative repair, development and proliferation of stem cells, and tissue regeneration.

Traditional vs. Functional Medicine

Pharmaceutical companies realize there are big profits to be made utilizing the science of Glycobiology to develop new drugs. They are spending billions of dollars to synthesize the sugars to add to the drugs, believing the drugs will work better.

Advancing diagnostics of glycans will enable scientists to better understand the composition of Smart Sugars and proteins.

In the future, in the traditional mode, most medical professionals will be educated by the drug companies on why they should be prescribing these drugs for their patients.

Functional medicine is the medical practice or treatments that focus on optimal function of the body and its organs, treating the whole system, not just symptoms, usually involving natural approaches.

The GLYCOSCIENCE INSTITUTE foresees Functional Medical physicians will use advanced Glycoscience Diagnostics to evaluate a patient's glycans that forecast what the patient's health will be years in advance. These diagnostics will guide clinics to understand what Smart Sugars are needed.

The GLYCOSCIENCE INSTITUTE teaches that Glycobiology helps people of all ages be healthier by improving the quality of the body's cellular communication system by naturally ncreasing the number of glycans.

The new era of medical exploration of the red planet reveals just how safe it can be when you obey the natural laws. Doctors and patients are learning about and advancing the power of Smart Sugars. Some scientists believe we can have an extended stay on the planet and be in good health for well over 100 years.

Glycoscience pioneers are making "proving ground" discoveries and designing advanced clinics to sustain life beyond normal expectancy and pave the way for future missions. The doctors and scientists of tomorrow will do what has never been done and go where no man has gone before. We learn from what we envision.

Innovative partnerships of doctors, businessmen, and scientists will blaze a trail for the people to follow. These trail blazers will achieve a satisfaction that few ever have... that of helping the human race know the possibilities of health.

Our teams are making it happen and many people will become a part of the team of their choice. Possibilities will be revealed to all who seek more knowledge. Experts from around the world are collaborating in disciplines of Glycoscience that the world knows little or nothing about.

The GLYCOSCIENCE INSTITUTE was designed to educate and partner with all those who are interested in going to another level of awareness and application. Everyone, regardless of their status or lot in life can benefit from the knowledge of Glycoscience.

We offer classes and private consultation in various disciplines of Glycoscience that will benefit every healthcare professional. Our desire is to better equip and empower doctors to be the best in their field. This is an exciting time to learn about the meticulous work your instructors have achieved in this technology and how Glycoscience will change the world.

Every medical student and pre-med student can benefit from classes at the GLYCOSCIENCE INSTITUTE because it will educate them in what we have learned over two decades and put into practice the knowledge that will help many. The student will learn from authorities in Glycoscience about the trends in healthcare and the future of medicine in detail that you never new was available. One of the biggest paradigm shifts is in its early stage. Those who have the knowledge and anticipate these changes will be better equipped to help their patients and the next generation. The student will gain authority to proceed in the many disciplines that are forging into mainstream medicine. Is there a disease, is there an ailment, that cannot be addressed with enhanced immunology? Is there a person on planet earth that cannot benefit from having a better understanding of Glycoscience?

Every person, sick or well, can benefit from these classes. We want to partner with individuals willing to learn and have the foundational belief of the Father of Medicine, Hippocrates, who said, *"First, do no harm."* Hippocrates believed that from conception to death that no life should be harmed. The Hippocratic Oath is not followed very well today from when he said, *"Let food be thy medicine and medicine be thy food."*

Report: Ongoing Research for Improving the Communication Receptor Sites on the Neurons:

Neurotransmitters are chemicals that help neurons communicate. As I have written throughout the book, glycosylation of the cells improves the neurotransmitters' ability to communicate more clearly and have amplified signals.

When various sugars are available in the body, the compounds or compositions may be useful as tissue protectants including neuroprotectants and cardioprotectants.

Cannabinoid receptors are transported by glycosylated proteins (glycoproteins) involved in transmitting and receiving data involved in physiological processes that include appetite, pain, pleasure, mood, and memory.

There has been much orchestrated confusion about hemp/marijuana cannabidiol (CBD) and tetrahydrocannabinol (THC). I am not a proponent of smoke or any carcinogen pumped into your lungs.

Hemp seed oil (CBD) is not psychoactive as is THC. CBD is antioxidant and neuroprotectant. The molecule appears the same but the bonding is different. The confusion is that in the laboratory two molecules appear to be identical but clinically they are worlds apart in function. We have found that a slight degree of difference in the bond of two atoms. In sugars, the bond provides a drastic difference in functionality. I have written much about this with the sugar Trehalose. While this may not be immediately visible to the eye, sometimes it is. Carbon is carbon but it can appear as coal or diamond.

Two major potential problems appears to be the legality and purity of the oil. Research will prove CBD to be rich in health benefits but a landmine of possible risks amplified by Big Pharma.

In the human body every atom, every molecule, in fact everything functions in collaboration with the Smart Sugars. The function of cannabinoid receptors transported by glycosylated proteins in the brain is determined by the purity of all the molecules. The tipping point is brilliance or madness.

Source and References:

Smart Sugars Lesson #77 http://www.endowmentmed.org/pdf/SmartLesson77

Chapter Four

Oxidation or Oxygenation

**Breathing oxygen is a
rather important factor in life.**

Breathing oxygen is a rather important factor in life. Researchers conclude that some twenty-five percent (25%) of the oxygen you breath is used by the brain.

Many significant studies have been conducted concerning neurological function and oxygen. Deep breathing exercise is a cost-free contribution to all health challenges and I highly recommend it for fibromyalgia and chronic fatigue.

Supporting the oxygenation process is a fibromyalgia research project conducted at Rice University in Houston in collaboration with institutes in Israel.

A clinical trial involving women diagnosed with fibromyalgia showed the painful condition improved in every one of the 48 who completed two months of hyperbaric oxygen therapy. Brain scans of the women before and after treatment gave credence to the theory that abnormal conditions in pain-related areas of the brain may be responsible for the syndrome.

Results of the study appeared in the open-access journal PLOS One.

Eshel Ben-Jacob was an adjunct professor of biosciences at Houston's Rice University, a senior investigator at Rice's Center for Theoretical Biological Physics and a professor of physics and member of the Sagol School of Neuroscience at Tel Aviv University. He was the lead author of the proof-of-concept study who developed the analytical method used to show the association between patients' improvement and changes in their brains.

Symptoms in about seventy percent (70%) of the women who took part in the study showed the most improvement with hyperbaric oxygen treatment where he found significant changes in their brain activity.

The study at Rice University and institutes in Israel showed patients in a small trial experienced remarkable improvement after two months of treatment. The Sagol School of Neuroscience at Tel Aviv University was involved. Patients were exposed to pure oxygen at higher-than-atmospheric pressures to push more oxygen into a patient's bloodstream for delivery to the brain.

One patient was an Oxford graduate student who had developed fibromyalgia after suffering a traumatic brain injury in a train crash. Often fibromyalgia is triggered by a traumatic event.

But by the end of treatment some of the women showed remarkable improvement, Ben-Jacob said.

The clinical trial involved 60 women who had been diagnosed with fibromyalgia at least two years earlier. A dozen left the trial for various reasons, but half of the 48 patients who completed it received 40 HBOT treatments five days a week over two months. The 90-minute treatments exposed patients to pure oxygen at two times the atmospheric pressure.

The other half were part of what Ben-Jacob called a crossover-control group. They were evaluated before the trial and after a control period that saw no improvement in their conditions. After the two-month control, they were given the same HBOT treatment as the first group and experienced the same relief, according to the researchers.

The researchers noted the successful treatment enabled patients to drastically reduce or even eliminate their use of pain medications. "The intake of the drugs eased the pain but did not reverse the condition, while HBOT did reverse the condition," the researchers wrote.

Efrati said the findings warrant further study. "The results are of significant importance since, unlike the current treatments offered for fibromyalgia patients, HBOT is not aiming for just symptomatic improvement," he said. "HBOT is aiming for the actual cause — the brain pathology responsible for the syndrome. It means that brain repair, including even neuronal regeneration, is possible even for chronic, long-lasting pain syndromes, and we can and should aim for that in any future treatment development."

Co-authors of the paper are Ham Golan, Olga Volkov, Gregori Fishlev, Jacob Bergan and Mony Friedman of the Sackler School of Medicine at Tel Aviv University and the Assaf Harofeh Medical Center, Zerifin, Israel; Yair Bechor of the Institute of Hyperbaric Medicine at Assaf Harofeh; Yifat Faran of Ashkelon Academic College, Israel; Shir Daphna-Tekoah of Ashkelon Academic College and Kaplan Medical Center, Israel; Gal Sekler of Tel Aviv University; Jacob Ablin of the Tel Aviv Sourasky Medical Center and Tel Aviv University; and Dan Buskila of Ben-Gurion University of the Negev, Israel.

http://news.rice.edu/2015/06/02/hyperbaric-hope-for-fibromyalgia-sufferers-2/

Read more at: http://news.rice.edu/2015/06/02/hyperbaric-hope-for-fibromyalgia-sufferers-2/#sthash.1lsmuK2S.dpuf

13 April 1952 - 5 June 2015
Following the fibromyalgia study Eshel Ben-Jacob died suddenly at his home in Israel June 5, 2015.

About the Author

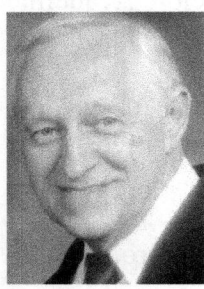 JC Spencer is the author of the Glycoscience Whitepaper and has written several Glycoscience books. He has studied the works of more than 700 M.D.s, PhDs, Scientists, Researchers, and Educators in the field of Glycoscience and brain function and collaborated with schools, universities, and research labs in thirteen countries. He has enjoyed international adventures and speaking engagements in many countries. Since the 1990s, he has worked closely with several specialists, doctors, and healthcare professionals in Glycoscience which resulted in the publishing of peer-reviewed papers evidencing improved brain function in Alzheimer's patients, and pilot surveys for various neurodegenerative challenges including Alzheimer's, Parkinson's, Huntington's, ALS, Lyme, Autism, and ADHD. He passionately envisions the field of QUANTUM GLYCOSCIENCE as the proven bull's eye, the Rosetta Stone, the Holy Grail, of medicine and of all healthcare.

JC Spencer is Founder and CEO of the TEXAS ENDOWMENT FOR MEDICAL RESEARCH, Inc, a 501(c)(3) faith-based medical research and education organization and think tank based in Houston, Texas. In collaboration with various organizations, he has conducted surveys on specific biological sugars throughout the United States, Canada, and some foreign countries. He has written extensively about Glycoscience and is also founder and CEO of the GLYCOSCIENCE INSTITUTE.

Mr Spencer and his wife, Karen, have four children, ten grandchildren and five great-grandchildren. They live in Houston, Texas.

Other books by the author are available on Amazon and elsewhere:

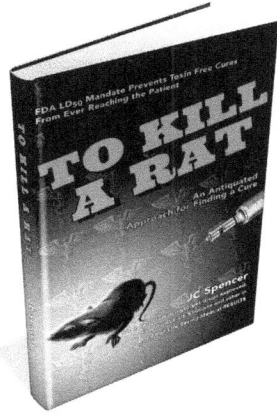

To Kill A Rat

True stories of hope where there was no hope. The book also reveals the secret of why the FDA requires a rat to die to develop a new drug.

http://tokillaratBOOK.com

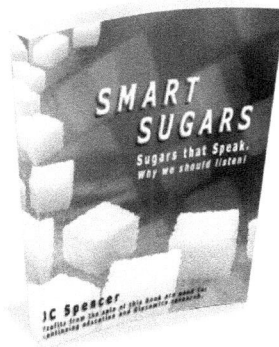

Available on Amazon and elsewhere in various formats including hard bound, paperback, audio, and Kindle.

For other books on Amazon, search:
Smart Sugars JC Spencer

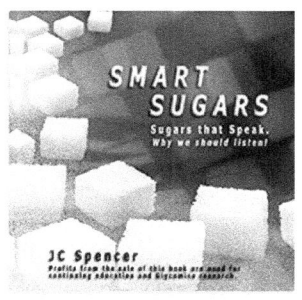

Listen to an audio sample of Smart Sugars on Amazon. Simple request:
Smart Sugars audio

www.ingramcontent.com/pod-product-compliance
Lightning Source LLC
Chambersburg PA
CBHW061452180526
45170CB00004B/1668